Vanishing Act

TRANSFORM YOURSELF LIKE NEVER BEFORE

BY HARSHITA BISHT

Introduction

THE POWER OF DISAPPEARING

In our constantly connected world, the idea of disappearing might seem strange, even counterintuitive. But within the concept of "disappearing" lies a powerful potential for growth. It's not about physically vanishing, but rather about stepping away from the noise – the expectations, anxieties, and routines that hold us back. It's a chance to hit pause, re-evaluate, and reconnect with our authentic selves.

I once felt creatively stagnant, suffocated by the pressure to constantly produce. So, I took a digital detox. I disappeared from social media, silenced notifications, and retreated to a quiet cabin in the woods. That week of disconnection was transformative. Away from the external noise, I rediscovered my passion for writing, explored new creative avenues, and returned feeling energized and inspired.

This experience forms the core of my book, "The Power of Disappearing." The book is divided into three sections. Part one explores the different ways we can "disappear" – from digital detoxes to solo travel, and even carving out sacred quiet time in our daily lives. Part two delves into the benefits of this temporary disconnect – increased focus, emotional clarity, and a deeper sense of purpose. Finally, part three equips readers with practical tools and strategies to implement "disappearing" practices into their lives, guiding them towards a more fulfilling and authentic existence.

Part 1

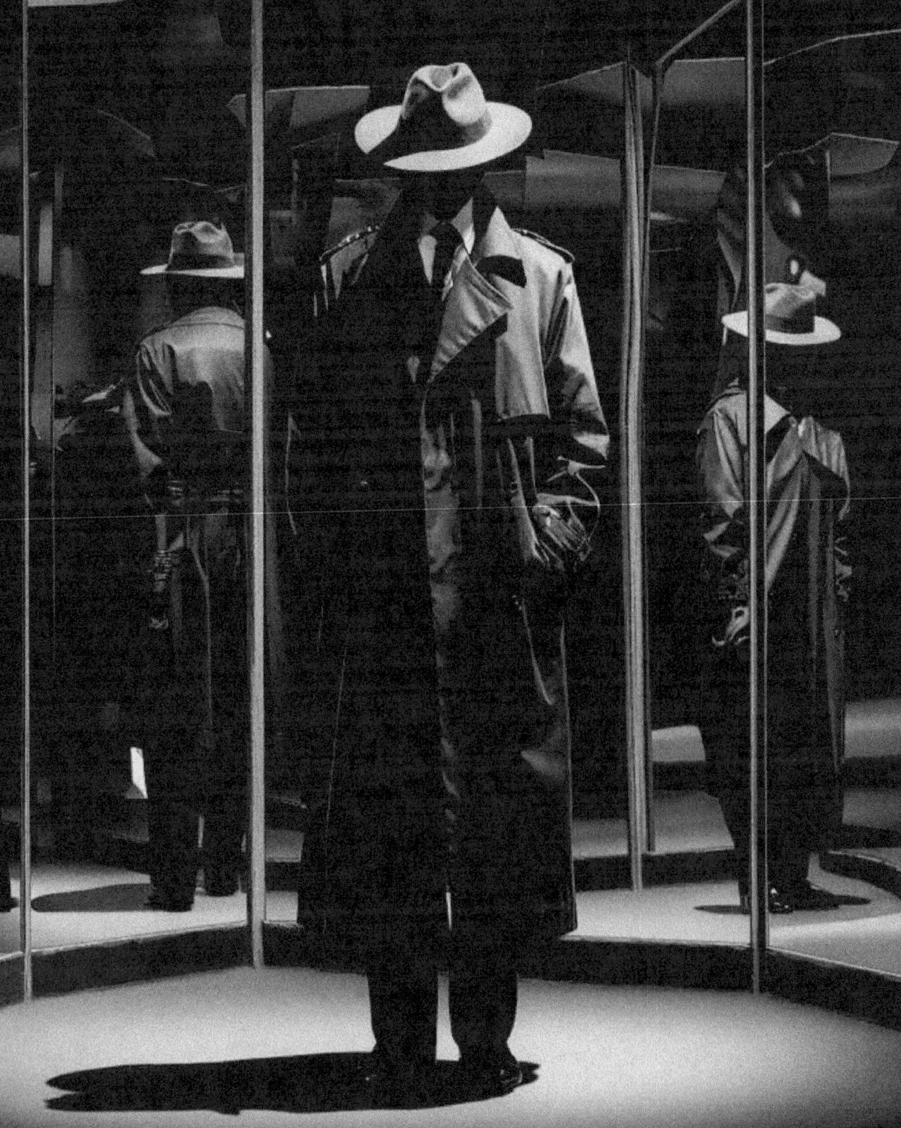

HOW TO DISAPPEAR

Chapter 1:

THE ART OF SILENCE

We all have that friend – the one who announces their goals from the rooftops, only to lose steam halfway through. In "Vanishing Act," we explore the power of silence, particularly in the early stages of transformation. This chapter delves into the importance of keeping your plans and progress a secret, even when the urge to share screams the loudest.

Why the Hush?

We often underestimate the power of external validation. When we broadcast our intentions, the pressure to conform to expectations can become overwhelming. Keeping things quiet allows us to focus on internal motivation, fostering a sense of ownership and autonomy over your transformation journey.

Taming the Share Button:

Let's face it, social media thrives on instant gratification. Resisting the urge to post about every step can feel unnatural. This chapter equips you with techniques to manage that urge. We'll explore strategies like delayed gratification, where you celebrate milestones privately before sharing them with the world.Additionally, you'll learn how to reframe your perspective – view silence not as suppression, but as a powerful tool for cultivating focus and determination.

Practice Makes Perfect:

Knowing the "why" is crucial, but so is the "how." Chapter 1 concludes with practical exercises to strengthen your restraint muscle. We'll explore techniques like journaling your progress instead of posting it, and identifying trusted confidantes who can offer support without judgment. By practicing these exercises, you'll build the discipline to leverage silence as a springboard for transformative change.

Chapter 2:

BECOMING A MYSTERY

Chapter 1 explored the power of cloaking your goals in silence. Now, we delve deeper into the transformative potential of strategic unavailability. In our hyper-connected world, this might seem radical, but within the act of disappearing lies a potent catalyst for change.

Why Disappear?

It's not about vanishing completely, but creating a sacred space for self-discovery. By becoming unavailable, you erect a boundary – not just with others, but with external pressures and distractions that derail progress. This focused inward journey allows you to explore desires, fears, and motivations with laser-like clarity.

The Power of Disappearing Acts:

History is peppered with examples of individuals who embraced unavailability for profound transformation. Think of Steve Jobs' pilgrimage to India, a period credited with shaping his revolutionary approach to technology.

Or J.K. Rowling, who found solace in solitary cafe sessions, birthing the magical world of Harry Potter. These "disappearances" fueled creativity and led to groundbreaking achievements.

Cultivating Your Mysterious Aura:

Fear not, becoming a mystery doesn't equate to social exile. This chapter guides you on cultivating a healthy dose of intrigue. You'll learn:

- The Art of Boundaries: Master the art of politely declining requests that don't align with your goals. Learn to say "no" with grace and finality.
- The Power of "Not Now": Prioritize your inner work without feeling obligated to explain your absence. Develop a "not now, but for a compelling reason" approach.
- Curating Your Digital Presence: Discover techniques to manage your online persona in a way that supports your transformation. Consider taking social media sabbaticals or limiting updates that don't reflect your new direction.

By embracing strategic unavailability, you cultivate fertile ground for self-discovery and personal growth. This chapter equips you with the tools to become a captivating "mystery" – unavailable to external distractions, but fully invested in the transformative journey within.

Chapter 3:

REPROGRAMMING YOUR MIND

Reprogramming Your Mind dives deep into the internal battle that can hinder transformation – the fear of judgment and the need for external validation. We explore the psychology behind social anxiety and how our desire for approval can hold us back. By understanding these mechanisms, you'll learn to detach from external opinions and trust your own inner compass.

This chapter equips you with practical exercises to build unshakeable self-confidence. You'll learn to identify and challenge the negative self-talk that can be our own worst enemy. We'll replace those inner criticisms with positive affirmations, reminding ourselves of our worth and capabilities. Visualization techniques will also be explored, allowing you to see yourself achieving your goals and celebrating milestones along the way. These exercises reinforce self-belief and fuel the motivation to keep moving forward on your transformative journey.

For a powerful dose of inspiration, Chapter 3 delves into a real-life case study. Take Maya, for example. A talented artist stifled by self-doubt, Maya constantly compared her work to others, leading to creative paralysis. After years of frustration, she decided to reprogram her mind. By identifying and challenging her negative self-talk ("My art isn't good enough"), Maya replaced it with affirmations ("I am a creative artist with a unique voice"). She visualized herself showcasing her art and embraced practices like daily sketching to celebrate small wins. The shift was remarkable. Maya rediscovered her passion for art, started exhibiting her work, and even garnered recognition from local galleries. Maya's story is a testament to the power of self-belief. By silencing her inner critic and focusing on her own journey, she unlocked her true artistic potential.

Chapter 4:

CRAFTING YOUR PERSONA

Chapter 4 of "Vanishing Act" takes a pivotal turn, shifting from shedding limitations to actively crafting your ideal future self. Entitled "Crafting Your Persona: Architecting Your Transformed Self," this chapter guides you on a journey of self-discovery and design.

Imagine the best version of you – confident, fulfilled, and thriving in all aspects of life. Visualization becomes your superpower here. Through guided exercises, you'll learn to paint a vivid mental picture of your ideal self. See yourself excelling in your career, radiating health and vitality, or navigating social situations with effortless ease. By anchoring these visualizations in your mind, you create a powerful roadmap for your transformation. This isn't just about daydreaming; it's about actively shaping the future you desire.

However, visualization is just the first step in crafting your persona. Chapter 4 delves deeper with introspective journaling prompts designed to solidify your identity and define your true goals. These prompts encourage you to explore the core values that define you, the activities that spark joy and fulfillment, and the impact you want to leave on the world. By answering these questions with honesty and introspection, you gain a crystal-clear understanding of the person you're striving to become. This newfound clarity becomes the foundation for your transformation journey. It acts as a guiding light, propelling you forward and ensuring your choices align with your ultimate vision for yourself.

PART 2

WHAT TO DO INE IN THE SHADOWS

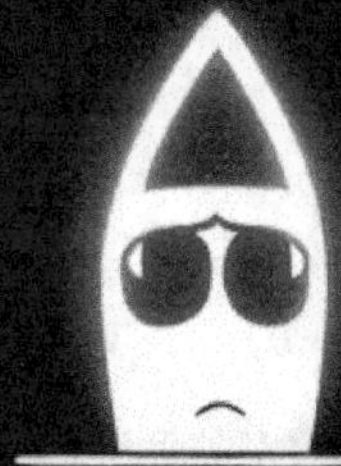

Chapter 5

SETTING AMBITIOUS PLANS

Chapter 5 of "Vanishing Act" takes your transformation journey from vision to action plan. Here, you'll conquer the art of setting clear, actionable goals that propel you forward.

The chapter dives deep into the SMART goal framework, ensuring your goals are well-defined and achievable. SMART stands for:

- **Specific**: Ditch vague goals like "get healthy." Instead, define a specific target, like "run a 5K race within 6 months."
- **Measurable**: How will you track progress? A measurable goal could be "reduce daily screen time by 30 minutes" or "lift 20 pounds more on my bench press by the end of the quarter."
- **Achievable**: Be ambitious, but realistic. Consider your current skills and resources when setting goals.
- **Relevant**: Align your goals with your overall vision. Does "running a marathon" fit your desire for better health, or would a different activity be more relevant?

Time-bound: Give your goals a deadline! A time-bound goal might be "learn the basics of a new language in 3 months" or "complete this online course by the end of the year."

By applying SMART, you craft goals that are clear, motivating, and achievable. Chapter 5 goes further, offering strategies to break down large goals into smaller, manageable steps. This keeps you focused and prevents feeling overwhelmed, ensuring you stay on track.

But setting goals is just the first step. Chapter 5 recognizes the importance of staying focused and motivated. Here are some key strategies:

- **Visualization Power**: Regularly revisit your visualizations from Chapter 4. Seeing your ideal self as the ultimate reward reignites motivation when faced with challenges.
- **Milestone Magic**: Break down large goals into smaller milestones. Completing these mini-goals fuels momentum and keeps you focused on the bigger picture.
- **Reconnect with "Why"**: Remind yourself of the deeper purpose behind your transformation. Reconnecting with your core motivations can rekindle your passion during setbacks.

Maintaining motivation is equally important. Chapter 5 offers practical tools:

- **Reward Yourself**: Celebrate milestones, big and small! Implement a reward system to acknowledge your progress. This positive reinforcement keeps you motivated and excited to continue.
- **Track Your Progress**: Seeing tangible evidence of your progress is incredibly motivating. The chapter provides downloadable worksheets designed to help you track your goals and milestones. Visually seeing your journey unfold reinforces your commitment and fuels your desire to keep moving forward.
- **Build Your Support System:** Surround yourself with positive and supportive individuals who believe in you and your goals. Chapter 5 encourages you to identify these individuals and leverage their encouragement to stay motivated throughout your transformation.

With these strategies and the downloadable worksheets, Chapter 5 equips you to not only set clear goals but also to maintain the focus and motivation required to achieve your transformative vision.

Chapter 6

THE POWER OF PROGRESS

While Chapters 4 and 5 of "Vanishing Act" focus on crafting your ideal self and setting goals, the journey doesn't end there. Transformation is a marathon, not a sprint, and Chapter 6 equips you with the tools to stay consistent, celebrate victories, and overcome obstacles.

The Power of Small Wins:

- **Celebrating Milestones**: Every step forward deserves recognition! Chapter 6 emphasizes the importance of acknowledging and celebrating small victories. This could be anything from completing a daily workout routine to mastering a new skill. Taking the time to celebrate reinforces positive behavior and keeps you motivated on your journey.
- **Tracking Progress**: Chapter 5 introduced downloadable worksheets for goal tracking. Chapter 6 encourages you to use these tools to not only track your progress towards major goals but also to celebrate smaller milestones along the way.

Seeing a visual record of your achievements fuels a sense of accomplishment and motivates you to keep going.

Staying Consistent:

- **Habit Building**: Transformation is about creating lasting change. Chapter 6 explores techniques for building positive habits that become an ingrained part of your lifestyle. This could involve setting daily reminders, finding an accountability partner, or rewarding yourself for consistent effort.
- **Schedule It In**: Treat your transformation like any important appointment. Chapter 6 suggests scheduling dedicated time in your calendar for activities that support your goals. This ensures these activities don't get squeezed out by the business of life

.

Conquering Obstacles:

- **Anticipate Challenges**: The road to transformation isn't always smooth. Chapter 6 encourages you to anticipate potential obstacles that might derail your progress. By identifying these challenges in advance, you can develop strategies to overcome them.
- **Develop Coping Mechanisms**: Life throws curveballs. Chapter 6 equips you with coping mechanisms to navigate setbacks and maintain your focus. This could involve relaxation techniques like meditation or journaling to process challenges and develop solutions.

\

Seek Support: Don't go it alone! Chapter 6 reminds you of the importance of your support system. Lean on friends, family, or mentors for encouragement and guidance during difficult times.

By incorporating these strategies, Chapter 6 empowers you to stay consistent, celebrate your achievements, and navigate any obstacles that may arise on your transformative journey.

Chapter 7

MAINTAINING SECRECY

Chapter 7 of "Vanishing Act" takes a surprising turn, diving into the concept of strategic secrecy. While the book promotes transformation, it challenges the idea that every detail needs to be shared. This chapter explores the power of keeping your plans hidden, particularly in the initial stages of your journey.

Here, you'll discover why discretion is a powerful tool. Sharing your goals with everyone can introduce external pressure and unsolicited advice, potentially leading to self-doubt and hindering progress. The chapter emphasizes the importance of intrinsic motivation – the internal drive that fuels your transformation. Keeping your plans hidden allows you to celebrate milestones internally, maintaining your focus and motivation without the need for external validation.

Chapter 7 also acknowledges the potential negativity from others. Not everyone will be supportive of your transformation, and negativity can be a significant obstacle. By keeping your plans private, you control your environment and minimize exposure to those who might discourage you. The chapter strengthens its argument with real-life success stories – individuals who achieved remarkable results by keeping their plans under wraps. Imagine a young entrepreneur who quietly honed a revolutionary idea, avoiding the naysayers who might have stifled their creativity. Their success story exemplifies the power of focused action in a protected space.

To help you cultivate this habit of discretion, Chapter 7 offers practical exercises. You'll learn to identify your inner circle – those trusted confidantes who will genuinely support you. The chapter equips you with techniques for politely declining discussions about your plans, offering vague responses or deflecting questions without revealing specifics. Finally, a "privacy audit" helps you take control of your online presence. This might involve making social media accounts private or limiting information about your goals.

By understanding the benefits of strategic secrecy and practicing these exercises, Chapter 7 empowers you to create a fertile ground for transformation, free from the noise and distractions of the external world. This allows your inner potential to flourish in a protected environment, paving the way for a successful and fulfilling transformation.

Chapter 8

DEALING WITH SETBACKS

The path to transformation in "Vanishing Act" is rarely a straight shot. Chapter 8 acknowledges the reality of setbacks and failures, but more importantly, equips you with the tools to navigate them with resilience. Here, you'll learn not just to handle these detours, but to emerge from them stronger and more determined.

Facing the Inevitable:

- **Normalizing Setbacks**: We all experience setbacks. Chapter 8 emphasizes that these are a normal part of the growth process, not a sign of personal failure. The key is to learn from them and use them as opportunities for improvement.

- **Reframing Failure**: Instead of viewing setbacks as the end of the road, the chapter encourages you to reframe them as valuable learning experiences. Analyze what went wrong. Did you underestimate the challenge? Did unforeseen circumstances derail you? Use this information to adjust your approach and ensure future success.

Building Resilience:

- **Developing Grit:** Chapter 8 highlights the importance of grit – the unwavering determination to see things through, even when faced with obstacles. The chapter offers strategies for cultivating grit, such as:
  - *Focusing on Long-Term Goals*: Keeping your ultimate vision in mind provides the motivation to push through temporary setbacks. Remind yourself of the "why" behind your transformation – the deeper purpose that fuels your journey.
  - *Embracing a Growth Mindset*: Believe that your abilities can be developed through effort. When faced with challenges, view them as opportunities to learn and improve.
- **Developing Coping Mechanisms**: Life throws curveballs. Chapter 8 equips you with coping mechanisms to navigate setbacks and maintain your focus. This could involve:
  - *Relaxation Techniques*: Techniques like meditation or deep breathing can help you process challenges calmly and develop solutions.
  - *Journaling:* Journaling your thoughts and feelings about setbacks can provide clarity and help you develop strategies for moving forward.

Finding Inspiration in Overcoming Challenges:
- **Stories of Resilience**: Chapter 8 features real-life stories of individuals who overcame significant setbacks on their path to transformation.
    - *The Comeback Athlete*: Imagine a star athlete who suffers a major injury. Devastated but not defeated, they use their grit and determination to recover and achieve even greater success. Their story exemplifies the power of resilience and the human spirit's ability to overcome adversity.
    - *The Rejuvenated Artist:* The chapter might also feature the story of a painter who loses their eyesight in an accident. Devastated but not defeated, they explore new techniques and rediscover their artistic voice in a completely new way. Their story highlights the power of adaptation and the ability to find new paths to fulfillment.

By incorporating these strategies and drawing inspiration from real-life examples, Chapter 8 empowers you to develop the mental fortitude necessary to navigate challenges and emerge stronger from setbacks. This resilience becomes a cornerstone of your transformative journey. Remember, every setback is an opportunity to learn, adapt, and ultimately, achieve your full potential.

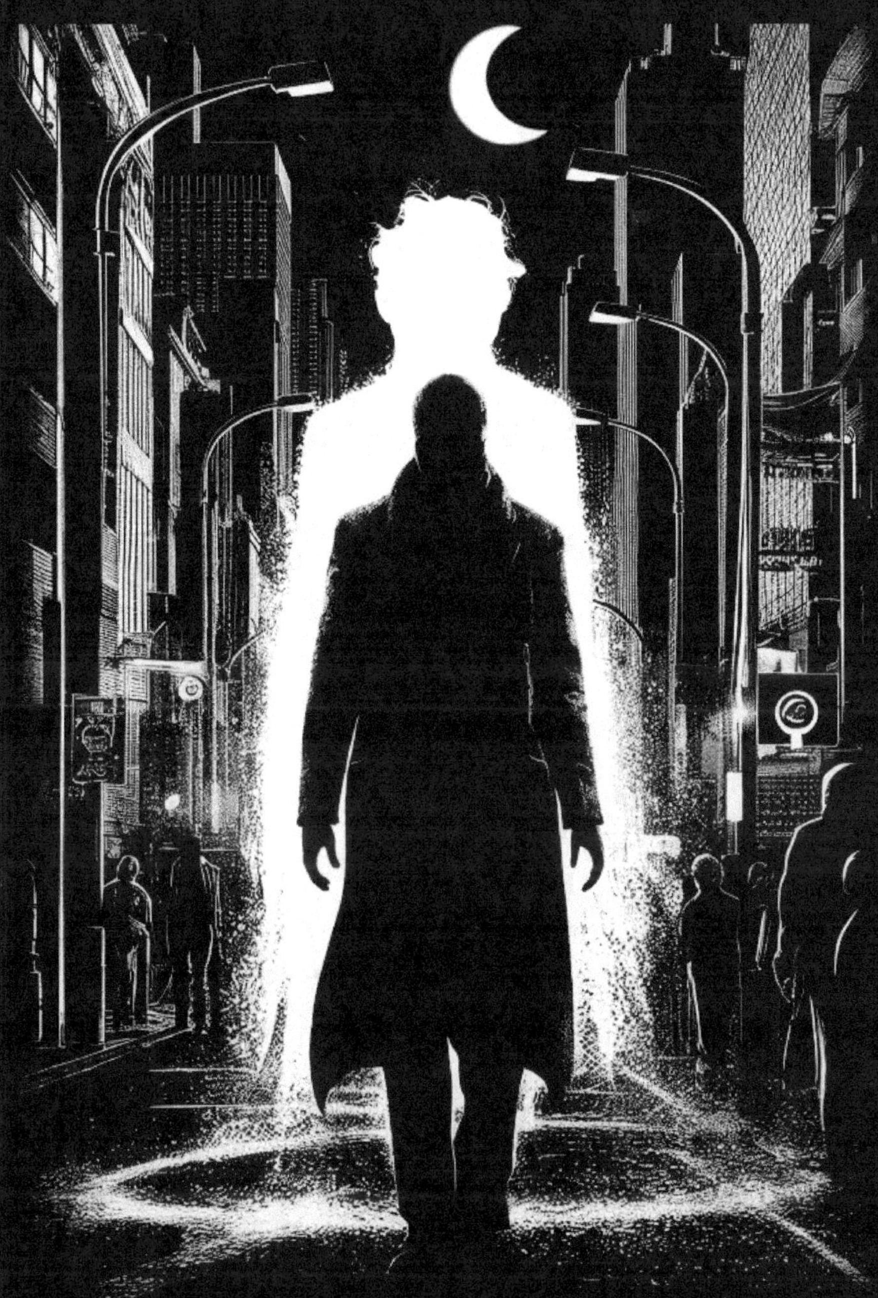
HOW TO
REAPPEAR
PART 3:

Chapter 9

PLANNING YOUR REAPPEARANCE

Chapter 9 of "Vanishing Act" marks a pivotal shift. Having cultivated your ideal self and navigated challenges, it's time to strategically re-enter the world. This chapter guides you on deciding when and how to unveil your transformation, maximizing its impact.

Knowing When to Re-emerge:

- **Confidence is Key**: Chapter 9 emphasizes the importance of confidence before re-emerging. Are you comfortable and proud of your transformation? Have you solidified your new identity and habits? Rushing the process can lead to feelings of vulnerability or inauthenticity.
- **Defining Your Goals**: Consider your reasons for re-emerging. Do you want to inspire others? Share your expertise? Re-entering the world with clear goals ensures your actions are aligned with your transformed self.

Strategies for a Grand Re-Entrance:
- **Curated Revelation**: Don't overwhelm your audience. Chapter 9 suggests a curated approach. This could involve sharing your story gradually, highlighting specific aspects of your transformation on social media or through carefully chosen conversations.
- **Action Speaks Louder**: Let your actions speak for themselves. Chapter 9 encourages you to showcase your transformation through your behavior and accomplishments. This could involve excelling at work, participating in activities that align with your new values, or radiating newfound confidence in your interactions.

Examples of Successful Re-appearances:
- The **Fitness** Influencer: Imagine a former couch potato who transformed into a fitness enthusiast. Their re-emergence might involve sharing their journey on social media, starting a blog to inspire others, or even participating in athletic events. Their success story demonstrates the power of transformation and motivates others to embark on their own journeys.
- The **Career** Changemaker: Chapter 9 might also explore the story of someone who left a high-paying but unfulfilling job to pursue their passion. Their re-emergence could involve starting a new business, showcasing their work at industry events, or even giving talks about their career transition. Their example highlights the courage it takes to prioritize fulfillment over societal expectations.

By following these strategies and drawing inspiration from real-life examples, Chapter 9 empowers you to orchestrate a re-emergence that not only celebrates your transformation but also inspires and motivates those around you. Remember, your re-appearance isn't just about you; it's about sharing the power of transformation with the world.

Chapter 10

CONTINUOUS IMPROVEMENT

"Vanishing Act" doesn't end with your grand re-emergence. Chapter 10 emphasizes that transformation is a lifelong journey. Here, you'll delve into the concept of continuous improvement, ensuring your growth never plateaus.

The Importance of Lifelong Learning:
- **Growth Mindset:** Chapter 10 reinforces the value of a growth mindset. Remember, your abilities and potential are not fixed. Embrace challenges as opportunities to learn and develop new skills.
- **Staying Curious**: Cultivate a sense of curiosity. The world is constantly evolving, and so should you. Chapter 10 encourages you to explore new ideas, interests, and experiences to keep your mind sharp and your transformation journey dynamic.

Techniques for Continued Growth:

- **Setting Stretch Goals**: Don't get complacent. Chapter 10 emphasizes the importance of setting ambitious yet achievable "stretch goals" that push you outside your comfort zone. This continuous goal setting keeps you motivated and ensures your transformation is a continuous process.
- **Seeking Feedback**: Nobody knows everything. Chapter 10 encourages you to seek constructive feedback from mentors, colleagues, or friends. This external perspective can highlight areas for growth you might have missed and help you refine your approach.
- **Embracing Feedback Loops:** Chapter 10 introduces the concept of feedback loops. Regularly evaluate your progress, identify areas for improvement, and adjust your strategies accordingly. This cyclical process ensures continuous refinement and propels you further along your transformative journey.

Exercises for Planning Future Growth:

- **Vision Board 2.0:** Revisit your vision board from Chapter 4. Has your ideal self evolved? Chapter 10 encourages you to create a new vision board that reflects your ongoing aspirations.
- **Future-Self Journaling**: Imagine yourself five years from now. Chapter 10 prompts you to journal about your goals, skills, and experiences in this future state. This exercise helps you identify the steps you need to take now to reach your future vision.

- **The Gratitude List**: Chapter 10 reminds you of the importance of gratitude. Regularly acknowledge your progress and celebrate your achievements. This fosters a positive mindset and fuels your motivation for continued growth.

By embracing these concepts and incorporating the practical exercises, Chapter 10 empowers you to approach transformation as a lifelong journey. You'll learn to view challenges as opportunities, continuously set goals, and refine your approach. Remember, the most important aspect of transformation is the act of continuous evolution. As you grow and learn, you'll keep "vanishing" your old self, unveiling a more empowered and fulfilling version with each step.

Chapter 11

EMBRACING THE SHADOWS

Chapter 11 flips the script. Transformation doesn't require a spotlight. It explores the value of quiet growth, fueled by introspection and purpose.

- **Inner Strength**: Chapter 11 highlights the power of introspection for self-discovery and authentic transformation.
- **Intrinsic Focus**: It revisits intrinsic motivation, where personal satisfaction drives your journey, not external validation.
- **Strategic Sharing:** Not all transformation requires secrecy. Share strategically with trusted confidantes for support or guidance.
- **Real-Life Examples:** The chapter showcases individuals who thrived in the shadows – anonymous philanthropists or unsung heroes who made a quiet but significant impact.

Chapter 11 empowers you to define your own path. Profound growth can occur quietly, driven by your own purpose. Embrace the shadows; transformation can be just as fulfilling there.

Chapter 12

LIVING YOUR NEW LIFE

Congratulations! You've transformed. Chapter 12 helps you fully embrace your new identity and navigate life as your best self.

Embracing Your Evolution:
- **Self-Acceptance:** Chapter 12 encourages you to fully accept your transformed self. Celebrate your achievements and own your new reality with confidence.

Maintaining Your Momentum:
- **Habit Reinforcement:** Chapter 12 emphasizes the importance of solidifying your positive habits. These habits are the foundation of your new life – regularly revisit the strategies from Chapter 5 to ensure they remain ingrained.
- **Growth Mindset Revisited:** Maintain a growth mindset. Chapter 12 reminds you that transformation is a continuous journey. Keep setting goals, seeking challenges, and learning new things.

A Final Note of Encouragement:

- **The Power Within:** Chapter 12 concludes by reminding you of the incredible power you hold. You have the ability to continuously transform and create the life you desire.

This chapter serves as a springboard, propelling you forward with the tools and confidence to live your best life, forever evolving as the empowered individual you've become.

Conclusion

Launch Your Transformation!

You've got the tools: setting goals, using secrecy, bouncing back from setbacks, and embracing lifelong learning. Now it's time to take action!

Key Takeaways:

- **Clear Goals**: Define your "what" with SMART goals.
- **Strategic Secrecy**: Focus on growth in a protected space.
- **Resilience is Key:** Learn from setbacks and emerge stronger.
- **Never Stop Growing**: Embrace challenges and continuous improvement.
- **Find Your Path**: Transformation can be loud or quiet – choose what fuels you.

Start Today!

- **Revisit Your Vision**: Reconnect with your ideal self for inspiration.
- **Set Small Goals**: Build momentum with achievable first steps.
- **Embrace the Journey**: It's a marathon, celebrate every win!

This book is your guide, but the adventure is yours. Transform into the incredible person you were meant to be!

thank you!